Learning to Lower
CHOLESTEROL

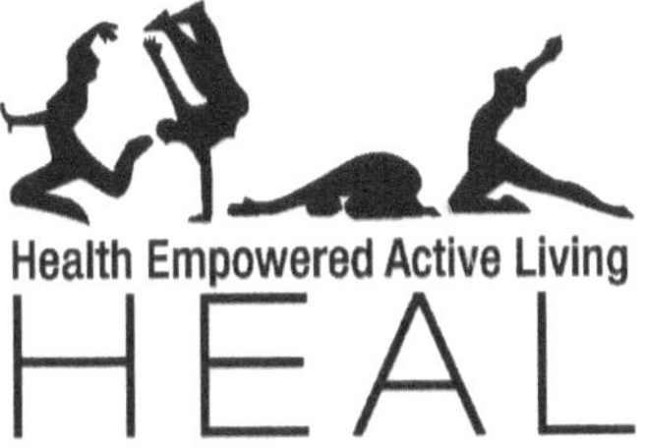

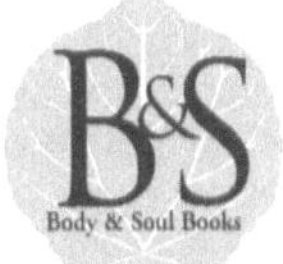

ISBN 978-93-81115-46-6

Design Mishta Roy
Layouts Ajay Shah
Printing Dhote Offset, Mumbai

Published in India 2011, by
BODY & SOUL BOOKS
an imprint of
LEADSTART PUBLISHING PVT LTD
Trade Centre, Level 1
Bandra Kurla Complex
Bandra (E), Mumbai 400 051, INDIA
T + 91 22 40700804
F +91 22 40700800
E info@leadstartcorp.com
W www.leadstartcorp.com

US Office
Axis Corp
7845 E Oakbrook Circle
Madison, WI 53717, USA

Disclaimer *The contents of this book do not purport to replace expert advice or obviate the role of the physician*

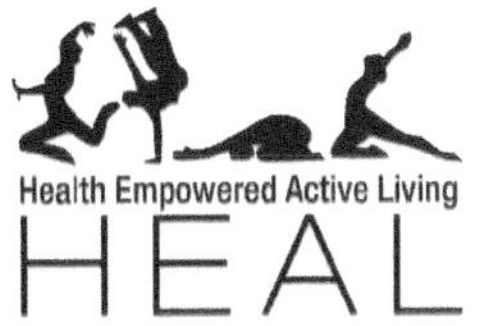

H E A L

ABOUT THE HEAL SERIES

As modern lifestyles move increasingly towards urban and urban-influenced living, our bodies too, face new and mutating challenges to cope with more processed food, less mobility, more time spent indoors in temperature controlled environments, less in green spaces and clean air, more exposure to television, computer, film and telephone screens and less to natural colours, sounds and sunlight. The natural way has become replaced by the artificial way, the instant recourse and quick-fix options.

In all ancient civilizations, stillness and peace were part of the way people lived, in harmony with the earth and nature. Now we have to go looking for it in spas and wellness farms. Stress has become ingrained in human endeavours. We have to consciously de-stress, meditate, do breathing exercises, in order to find equilibrium. What we once accepted as a natural process of fitness and living, is now a search and challenge for health empowerment.

But one thing has not changed – that good health remains the cornerstone of living life to its potential. Only the way in which we seek that elusive grail has changed. And yet, the core truths of health and healing remain the same, based on the five senses: Sight, Smell, Taste, Touch and Hearing. To these five is added one more: Silence – the art of being centred in stillness, where and when mind and being are in harmony.

This series of books has been developed to create holistic health consciousness and education in order to empower strong, active and fulfilled lives. Health remains the foundation on which we build our achievements, both collective and individual. These books are to meant to give laypeople a basic understanding of various ailments and diseases, as well as indicate the solutions available to them. The books do not seek to replace expert advice or the role of the physician.

To be informed is to be empowered. Decision-making and actions flow from knowledge, not general opinion or ignorance. To accept the challenges of our own health in an era of dynamic change all around – that is the ultimate goal.

ॐ

CONTENTS

CONTENTS

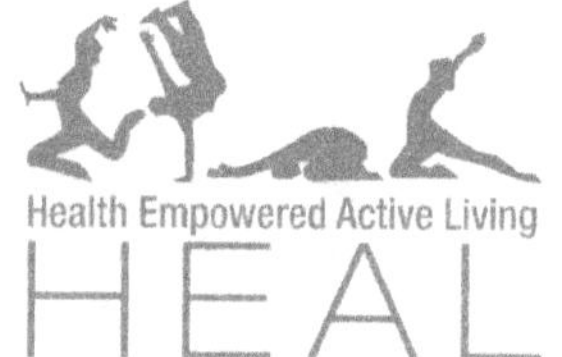
Health Empowered Active Living
HEAL

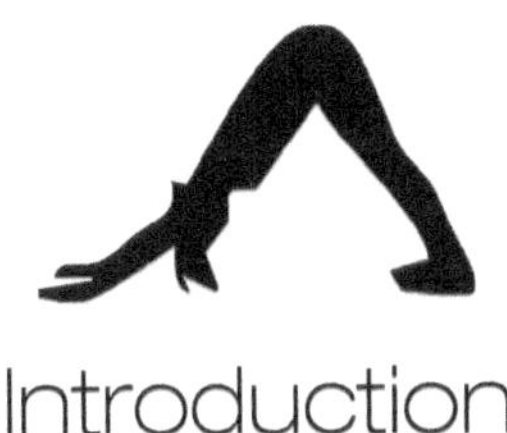

Introduction

Lowering Cholesterol Levels: Your Best Bet For A Healthy Future

The word 'cholesterol' comes from the Greek words *chole-* (bile) and *stereos* (solid), added to the suffix *-ol* (alcohol). François Poulletier de la Salle first identified cholesterol in solid form in gallstones, in 1769. However, it was only in 1815, that a chemist named Eugène Chevreul, actually named the compound 'Cholesterine'.

Cholesterol affects the human body in an adverse manner. This is a well known fact today. Lipoprotein is an assembly of proteins and lipids that carry cholesterols between the liver and the body tissues. Low density lipoprotein carrying cholesterol to the cells gets deposited on the artery walls, hardening them. Hence it is called 'bad cholesterol'. This hardening obstructs the smooth flow of blood and causes the status of the atherogens of the blood vessels to be ruined resulting in various diseases.

Contrary to popular belief, cholesterol is not completely bad for health. The value of this waxy substance that is non-soluble, is not widely known. Building membranes, nerve sheaths and cell walls, manufacture of bile, and production of hormones, are all aided by cholesterol. However, being exposed to high levels of it can cause various diseases. Hypertension is one of the main cardiovascular disorders caused by cholesterol. Sometimes, this can even be fatal. It can also lead to fibrosis and atherosclerosis, which is the dumping of extra fibre and fatty substances in the arteries.

Proper eating habits and regular exercise are the most effective ways of keeping cholesterol under check while over indulgence, bad diet and wrong lifestyles, can and do increase the cholesterol levels of the human body.

The best dietary practices for a cholesterol-trouble-free life

✓ Planning an entire week's menu in advance to ensure it is cholesterol-free and supplementing it with vegetables and fruits filled with fibres. Organic foods are much healthier as they do not have the chemicals that can trigger increased cholesterol levels. Complex carbohydrates of high standards should be used.

✓ People diagnosed with LDC should avoid egg yolk and eat more egg whites. Using whole wheat to prepare baked food stuffs and cereals for noodles, is also highly effective in reducing cholesterol levels. Refined sugar should be avoided as it contains a number of chemicals used in processing it so that the end product is fine and white. Unrefined sugar is less of a health hazard.

✓ Drink lots of water. It helps digestion, cleanses the body to maintain proper blood flow and maintains equilibrium in the body.

✓ Artificially made foods contain colouring agents, extenders and various additives. Hence they should be avoided. Instead, eat more root vegetables.

✓ Commercially made soft drinks contain large amounts of sugar, additives and artificial colours that can cause high cholesterol levels. Even chocolate beverages, other chemical drinks and caffeinated drinks like coffee, cause risk of high cholesterol levels. These should be replaced with fresh fruit juices for a healthier diet.

Food processing and baking usually include the usage of hydrogenated and trans-fats. These are highly destructive, even more than saturated fats produced from the same oils as them. Various palm oils, including olive oil, are the healthiest oils and help in lowering cholesterol levels of the entire family. Even though they are expensive, they can help in warding off various diseases caused by other oils.

High cholesterol levels can cause strokes or hypertension, both of which can even be fatal. These risks can be avoided by keeping in tune with your body with regular check-ups so that in case of high cholesterol levels, effective steps can be taken to reduce it before it is too late.

৪০৫৪

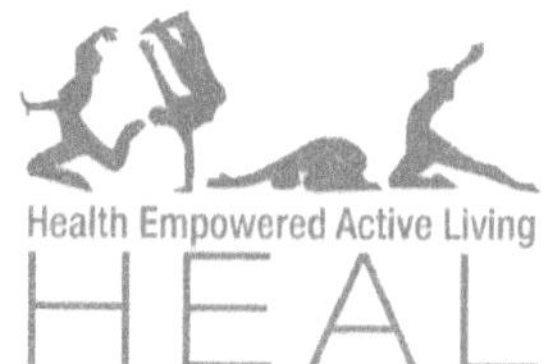
Health Empowered Active Living
HEAL

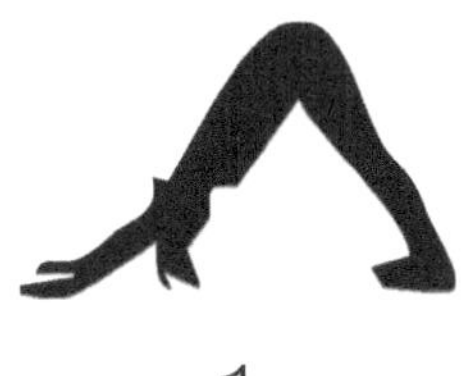

1

CHOLESTEROL LEVELS
Readings, Risks & Control

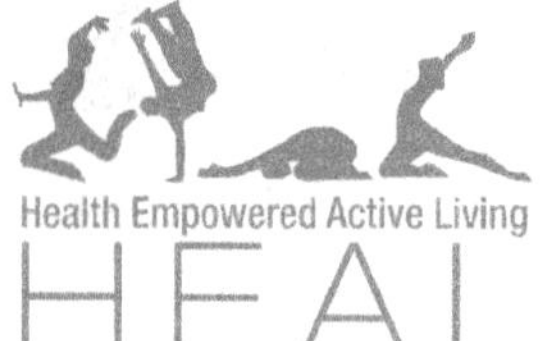

UNDERSTANDING CHOLESTEROL LEVELS

More than half of the world's population today has high cholesterol. What this means is that every other person that you see walking down the street is at risk for some sort of heart disease. The average person does not even know where their cholesterol levels stand, since you cannot see or feel high cholesterol. However, the statistics speak for themselves; you need to understand cholesterol in order to be able to deal with it. Once you get past the code, it is fairly simple to comprehend.

There are actually five different ways which you can use to get a complete reading on your own cholesterol levels and these are:
- total cholesterol levels
- HDL
- LDL
- total/HDL ratio
- LDL/HDL ratio

These measurements are actually written down to be what is desirable and what is not desirable.

Measurement units for checking cholesterol are conducted as milligrams per deciliter. It is extremely confusing if you try to look at these separately. You can talk to your doctor if you really want to understand your cholesterol levels and what, if anything, you need to do about them or how to maintain them properly.

Here are the actual numbers that are involved when it comes to your cholesterol:

- overall desired level............below 200 mg/dL
- borderline level...................200 to 240
- total risk...........................above 240

This is just for your overall levels. When it comes to breaking it down to each individual level, your doctor can best explain those to you.

Explaining HDL Cholesterol

When you think of your cholesterol, chances are all you care about is that it is low, but HDL levels are not the same as general cholesterol levels. It is actually just a section of your overall cholesterol when it comes to your HDL levels you actually want to be high. HDL is not the same as cholesterol in any way. In fact, your HDL levels are high density lipoproteins. We need lots of these. Their role in our body is to carry cholesterol away from the body as soon as LDL has brought it.

There are several different ways that you will want to achieve this. On the list are: excessive smoking, alcohol, body weight, exercise and medications. Let us look at the actual numbers on this. You have to remember that the smallest changes in HDL levels are significant. It would be going too far to say it is exponential, but a 1 mg/dL increase in your HDL cholesterol levels means as much as a 2 to 4 percent reduction in risk of heart disease and cardiac problems in general.

Knowing that your HDL levels need to be high is one thing. Here are the actual figures to explain. Your numbers are too low if they are at 37 mg/dL for men and at 47 mg/dL for women. The normal range for men to have is about 40 to 50 mg/dL, and for women 50 to 60 mg/dL. This is a concern as many people get these levels backward. It helps if you try to see a reasonable goal which would be to increase your HDL cholesterol levels by 10 mg/dL from whatever it is now, since most of us need more than what we have.

৪৩০৪

THINGS THAT WILL GIVE YOU HIGH CHOLESTEROL

By now, you probably know a lot about the risks of heart disease; especially with the vast amount of information that is available on this subject. However, you should also know that there are many different risk factors for high cholesterol that we never seem to pay enough attention to. What are they? What do they have to do with you? The first thing that needs to be said, however, that much of what follows may seem like plain common sense! And yet, half of all people either suffer or are at risk from, cholesterol-related disease.

Some of the foods that can contribute to your high cholesterol are fast foods, chips, soft drinks, candy bars, refined sugars, butter cream, fried cheese, fried dough, and cotton candy. These are the ones you can control by simply not eating them whenever possible. They are familiar, the kinds of comfort food that most of us have been eating since we were children. However, you should be warned that they will kill you if you let them so it stands to reason that your health compels you to avoid them. Some risk factors for high cholesterol are part of your normal everyday lifestyle.

Weight problems, smoking, alcohol abuse, all tend to stem from daily life routines and habits. Some of the causes of high cholesterol cannot be prevented. For example, when it is hereditary. Diabetes, kidney disease, liver disease, hyperthyroidism are just some of the dangers that these foods can cause; high cholesterol is just another side-effect.

₧₧

CHOLESTEROL READINGS EXPLAINED

It is highly recommended that one gets cholesterol levels checked once every few months. The cholesterol reading received will basically consist of:

- the total level of cholesterol
- level of lipoproteins
- triglycerides
- levels of lipoprotein cholesterol (high density)

This report will enable the physician to get a basic overall view of your health. If your physician needs different levels checked which gives a combinable reading, it is a splendid idea if one has the three levels of cholesterol (which are nothing but the sum of the cholesterol, LDL cholesterol and HDL), regularly monitored and verified.

The optimal range of total cholesterol is around 200mg to 239mg with 200mg being the spot on value. Researchers have predicted that one is at a risk of attack or any other heart disease if the total reading is above 240mg.

Low Density Lipoprotein Cholesterol

LDL form of cholesterol is the kind one must avoid, in other words the bad one. This type of cholesterol increases the risk of heart diseases by blocking the arteries with deposits of cholesterol. Hence, having levels of bad cholesterol which tend to be on the higher side, is bad for the body.

- The ideal limit of LDL level of cholesterol is 200 milligrams.
- The optimum range being 200-240 milligrams.
- Above that is potentially dangerous.

High Density Lipoprotein Cholesterol

LDL form of cholesterol is the kind one can call the 'good' cholesterol. Let us look into why it is considered good. What basically happens is that HDL transfers the surplus cholesterol to the liver from the tissues. This is converted to bile in the liver by breaking it down.

- The ideal limit of HDL level of cholesterol is 40 milligrams.
- The optimum range being 40-45 milligrams.
- Above 60 milligram protects ones heart and improvises on the brain's routines which manage the blood vessels.

Triglycerides

Triglycerides are nothing but a kind of fat. It accumulates in the body as fat and then slips into the blood stream. These constitute most of the fats in one's diet.

These harmless looking triglycerides are some of the prime contributors to heart disease. In the higher ranges of dose, it is known to thicken the blood arteries which may lead to a stroke or heart attack or any other kind of heart disease.

- The optimum range of triglyceride is between 150 and 199 milligrams.
- Not exceeding 200 milligrams.

There is actually nothing called an ideal reading. It differs from person to person depending on numerous factors. If the readings are pretty high a change in lifestyle is recommended. One must make maintain a healthy lifestyle to live a long life.

৪০৫৪

MEASURING CHOLESTEROL

Cholesterol Basics
According to statistics put out by the American Heart Association, over half the American population have less than desirable cholesterol levels. But how do we know how grave those risks are when we are seeing a reflection of ourselves? These numbers help the average person to understand the gravity of the risks and because of this, makes it easier to establish achievable goals.

Measuring Your Own Cholesterol Levels
There are actually five different ways to measure for a complete reading on your cholesterol levels:
- total
- HDL
- LDL
- total/HDL ratio
- LDL/HDL ratio

These measurements are actually categorized as desirable, borderline, and of course, at-risk. Measurement units are milligrams per deciliter. It is extremely misleading to consider any of them on their own. Consult your doctor to best understand your cholesterol levels and what, if anything, to do about them or how to maintain them properly.

Here is how it really works in terms of numbers.
- Total desirable.....................below 200 mg/dL
- Total borderline level...........200 to 240
- At-risk level.........................above 240
- HDL ideal level....................above 45 mg/dL
- HDL borderline level...........35 to 45

- HDL at-risk level.................below 35
- LDL ideal level....................below 130 mg/dL
- LDL borderline level.............130 to 160
- At-risk LDL level.................above 160
- Total/HDL ideal ratio is........below 4.5
- Total/HDL borderline...........4.5 to 5.5
- At-risk total/HDL.................above 5.5
- LDL/HDL ideal ratio............below 3
- LDL/HDL borderline............3 to 5
- At-risk LDL/HDL.................above 5

Those are a lot of numbers! What they show is that one very important set of numbers that you should bear in mind, is that every milligram per deciliter, makes a very large difference: with a 10 mg/dL drop in your overall cholesterol, comes an approximate 40 percent decrease in risk of heart disease. Is that not a good enough reason for you to want to do something about it?

When it comes to actually doing something about your cholesterol levels, a balanced diet, combined with a good fitness regimen is your best bet in combating high cholesterol. You have to be both active and eat right to maintain the right balance. You can look to the charts later in the book, as a means of being sure that your eating habits are balanced. Supplements of vitamins will not be able to compensate for your poor eating. You have to eat whole foods for any of this to be effective, and you must stay off heavy, fatty, junk foods to keep your cholesterol balanced.

୫୬ଠ୫

HDL CHOLESTEROL LEVEL

What is HDL Cholesterol Level?
When you think of cholesterol, your only thought is that it should be lower. However, HDL levels are not the same. The higher the better, is the necessary information when it comes to HDL cholesterol levels. HDL is not the same as cholesterol. In fact, your HDL levels are high-density lipoproteins. Our bodies can never seem to have quite enough of them. Their role in the body is to carry cholesterol away from body tissues, after LDL has carried it to them. Because LDL vastly outnumbers HDL by about 3 to 1, we are much better off if we can raise our HDL cholesterol levels.

There are several different ways to achieve this. On the list are to cut out excessive smoking, alcohol, body weight, exercise and medications. Let us look at the actual numbers on this. You have to remember that the smallest changes in HDL levels are significant. It would be going too far to say it is exponential, but a 1 mg/dL increase in your HDL cholesterol levels means as much as a 2 to 4 percent reduction in risk of heart disease and cardiac problems in general.

Breaking Down the Numbers on HDL Cholesterol Levels
When we start thinking about HDL levels, you need to remember that the numbers are different for men and women. In general, the average figure for HDL is approximately 40 mg/dL for what someone wants in HDL cholesterol levels. That is certainly the range that you have to think in terms of.

At this point we should go from risky HDL to average HDL to ideal HDL levels. The too-low danger flag about this goes out at 37 mg/dL for men and at 47 mg/dL for women. The normal range for men to have is about 40 to 50 mg/dL, and for women 50 to 60 mg/dL. The general target range for HDL cholesterol levels, but you have to remember that nothing is set in stone in this area, but it is about 60 mg/dL. A reasonable goal we can all set is and should be to increase HDL cholesterol levels by 10 mg/dL from whatever it is now.

As you can see, there is a vast difference from your cholesterol levels and your HDL levels. It is wise for you **not** to confuse the two of them. Commonsense would be for you understand that HDL levels work in the exact opposite manner that cholesterol does However, your HDL levels are akin to monitoring your cholesterol in that they both play huge roles in your overall health.

It is amazing how many people get so involved in their cholesterol levels that they forget about everything else! But the simple truth is, you can keep your HDL levels in within regulation figures simply by eating a balanced and nutritious combination of whole foods.

శుభం

CONTROLLING YOUR CHOLESTEROL

How to best control it if you have high cholesterol, depends on how high it is and why it is so high in the first place. By doing this research, you will at least be aware of the risk of having high cholesterol. You may already know that you have it but may just want to learn more about it. Either way, you will need to get a grip on your cholesterol and get informed about controlling it.

You may know that cholesterol plays a significant and decisive role in triggering heart disease. The primary causes of heart attack and stroke are clogged arteries and blood clots. The arteries travel to the heart or the brain and high cholesterol is what clogs these vital arteries. This is the main reason whu it is important to control high cholesterol before it gets to at-risk levels.

If you have high cholesterol, you will want to lower it. If you do not have high levels, you still want to know how to avoid it in the first place. Your first step to controlling high cholesterol is to establish healthy eating habits, healthy exercise habits and healthy drinking and smoking habits.

Healthy smoking habits are not smoking cigarettes and cigars that are considered light. Tobacco smokers have a single advantage over non-smokers: if they quit, they raise their HDL cholesterol levels very quickly, and that is a good thing. Healthy drinking habits are a little less crazy than smoking. Indications today state that a glass of red wine a day actually helps raise HDL cholesterol.

Healthy exercise habits mean regular aerobic exercise at least several times a week. This can be walking for 30 minutes, tennis, running, cycling, volleyball – whatever you enjoy doing and gives you a good cardiovascular workout. Healthy eating habits are one of the best ways to control high cholesterol. If you do this it will give you higher HDL and more importantly, much lower LDL. Place more emphasis on whole foods, fruits, vegetables, whole grains, legumes and less on animal products that are high in saturated fats. And focus less on processed foods. Maintaining your body properly means having a strong heart.

਼ੀ

CHOLESTEROL & YOUR LIFESTYLE

Cholesterol is produced in our bodies by the liver – the organ that uses the fats in our diet as fuel. What it produces is all the cholesterol the body needs to keep us moving. Why does it need cholesterol you may wonder? Among other things, it works by producing bile that is needed to help with digestion, protecting nerve fibres, building cell membranes, creating hormones, and also creating vitamin D.

Cholesterol that is found in our foods comes only from animal products that are rich in saturated fats. Plant foods have no cholesterol in them at all. Our bodies need fats of course, and we get a natural mix of them in many whole foods. But a diet that is too rich in saturated fats and trans-fatty acids such as those that you get in processed foods, is a proven health risk. Studies now indicate that polyunsaturated and monounsaturated fats, which can be found in olive and fish oils, are better for us and can help lower cholesterol.

Dietary fats are a concentrated source of special calories and because of this, form one of the two main causes of people being overweight and for obesity. Lack of exercise is the other reason for this. Decreasing dietary fat and increasing regular exercise are the first and quite frankly the easiest, steps that you can take to lower cholesterol and improve the health of your heart, as well as your overall well-being.

೮⦿ೞ

THE DEADLIEST EXCESS SUBSTANCE THAT COULD FORM IN THE BODY

The sustenance of outer membrane cells in every vertebrate requires cholesterol. It helps in blood circulation to the tissues of the body and blood plasma carried as alcohol and fatty lipids (steroids). Proper maintenance of cholesterol levels is necessary for unhindered flow of blood and plasma. The required levels of cholesterol should be maintained and should not be exceeded.

In today's world, fast foods and highway eateries are taking over the food market. Hence there needs to be awareness about the intake of additional or unwanted cholesterol that can affect health adversely. First of all proper awareness of the working of cholesterol and its effects on the metabolic process of the human body is necessary before knowing how to eliminate it. 'Bad cholesterol' refers to low-density lipoproteins. Lipoproteins are the carrier molecules. LDL can deposit cholesterol on the artery walls increasing its thickness and thus obstructing normal passage of blood. This causes arthrosclerosis. On the other hand, high density lipoproteins are the 'good cholesterols'.

The various functions of good cholesterol includes: manufacturing of bile, anti-oxidants, digestion of fats that are essential for the function of vitamins like vitamin A, D, E and K, which are fat soluble. These vitamins help in various metabolic processes of the reproductive organs starting from puberty onwards right up until old age that depend on estrogen levels in the body.

The Good Cholesterol in Our Bodies Come from Two Sources
Almost 75%, that is three fourths, of the required good cholesterol

is produced in the body itself in the tissues of various organs like the liver, reproductive organs central nervous system, including the spinal chord and the brain, atheroma and adrenal gland. Any degenerative change in the atheroma can cause the development of coronary artery disease and atherosclerotic plaques that can hinder blood flow. This sudden clogging of the arteries can affect the flow of blood to and from the heart, resulting in heart attacks that can be fatal.

The rest of the cholesterol, that is 25%, comes from external sources. Hence one has to be aware of what one eats and to maintain a proper diet. Animal meat, dairy products and egg yolk contain large amounts of cholesterol. The amount of cholesterol intake must be carefully monitored as even a small excess can cause an imbalance of cholesterol levels in the body.

More than the Required 25% Cholesterol Can be Lowered

Use non-saturated cooking oils that can reduce the intake of fats. The healthiest oil containing non-saturated fats is olive oil, which is a palm oil. Others such as coconut oil, contain highly saturated fats. Eating fruits and vegetables with high fibre content, taking low sodium content foods and complex carbohydrates, can all greatly reduce cholesterol levels of the body. Soybeans, nuts, corn, wheat, legumes and staple cereals, are some of the best cholesterol reducing food stuffs.

Eating in restaurants and fast food eateries should be avoided as they contain high sodium content foods and saturated fats. Alcohol can also cause increase in cholesterol levels and should be avoided.

Omega-3 acids found in Mackerel, Salmon, some species of Tuna and deep sea fish, help in decreasing levels of idle cholesterol in the body.

Medicines, including reductase inhibitors such as HMG-COA, atorvastatin (Liptor) and lovastatin (Mevacor), which are statins, can be taken to effective reduce LDL but only with the guidance of a physician.

৪০৩

RISK FACTORS FOR HIGH CHOLESTEROL

With all the information available on cholesterol, you may consider yourself well-informed on the risks of heart disease. But in fact, the risk factors for high cholesterol are a completely different story. The first thing is to identify what the risks are.

Some risks are part of your diet such as fast foods, chips, soft drinks, candy bars, refined sugars, butter cream, fried cheese, fried dough, and cotton candy. These are the ones you can control with a great deal less effort than you think. You probably grew up eating these things. They are familiar to you and they are likely your comfort foods. However, you should be warned that they will kill you if you let them.

Some risk factors for high cholesterol are part of your normal everyday lifestyle. Weight problems, smoking, alcohol abuse, and laziness, all contribute to your daily life structure. Some of these are health conditions you did not choose for yourself. However, whether lifestyle driven or genetic, they are there and can destroy you. Diabetes, kidney disease, liver disease, hyperthyroidism are just some of the dangers that these foods bring in their delicious train.

Some specific prescription drugs can also destroy you. Blood pressure medicine (such as clonidine and methyldopa), diuretics (water pills), anabolic steroids, beta blockers, and progestins can all cause harmful or even fatal complications. All these risk factors for high cholesterol affect you in different ways but all of them are detrimental to your good health. If you take prescribed medications for other conditions, you should consult your doctor.

If you want to do something about the risks you face you must first be honest with yourself about what your problem areas are and face them. This may sound completely obvious to you already, but self-denial is a powerful force. If your diet is too heavy in saturated fats and transfatty acids, you will need to reduce them dramatically. If you do not exercise regularly, you should start because it is never too late. It does not have to be two hours at the gym every day, just a 30-minute walk will suffice. The most important thing is to face the risks and then deal with them.

Lowering your cholesterol does not have to be the most difficult thing you do, it is necessary only that it be a priority. In lowering your cholesterol, you are guaranteeing that you are working to prevent serious illnesses. You cannot always stop them altogether but you can combat them.

ᔆᔆ

SORTING FACT FROM FICTION ABOUT CHOLESTEROL

You will notice there is a great deal of confusion regarding cholesterol due to the fact that there seem to be too many kinds! Then there is the good cholesterol and the bad cholesterol. The average person is at a loss, unsure of what all the terms mean. But information is wealth and one must learn to distinguish between what is the truth about cholesterol and what is not.

Fact or Fiction?
Since I hardly ever fall ill and I'm an exercise freak, there is no way I can have cholesterol problem.

Here is the hard fact: if a person has very high cholesterol, he will not exhibit any of the symptoms of cholesterol. Exercising regularly is definitely a very good habit but it is not a sure shot prevention for cholesterol problems. It depends on a variety of factors like the food intake, gender, one's weight, family history and age.

Fact or Fiction?
It's generally old people who have high cholesterol levels.

This is definitely a myth. One can be young and still have high cholesterol levels. It is highly recommended that one gets cholesterol checked regularly. If heart diseases run in your family history or you have an unhealthy diet or live a very sluggish lifestyle, be alert. Cholesterol levels must be tested at regular intervals to keep complications at bay.

Fact or Fiction?
Intake of anti-oxidants like Vitamin C and Vitamin E ensures that one doesn't have any cholesterol problems.

Myth! Fiction! The intake of anti-oxidants may be help reduce the risk but do not ensure prevention as such. A combination of factors affects the cholesterol level. A healthy and balanced diet with a regular exercise regime helps reduce high cholesterol levels.

Fact or Fiction?
Red wine is good for keeping cholesterol down.

Red wine in meager amounts is known to increase HDL. But this has side effects. Red wine is high in calories and causes increase of triglycerides. This pressurizes the liver and increases blood pressure.

Fact or Fiction?
When buying any product, check for those that have low cholesterol level.

Fiction! Though some products may seem safe, behold, products which are low in cholesterol need not necessarily have low fat content too!

Fact or Fiction?
One must never attempt to lower one's cholesterol level.

The human liver naturally produces the amount of cholesterol required to perform the necessary functions. A non-sedentary lifestyle with a healthy diet will definitely enable one to reduce cholesterol levels.

Fact or Fiction?
Overweight people are more prone to high cholesterol levels.

This may be a contributing factor but not necessarily a definite one. As mentioned earlier, if one has high cholesterol, the symptoms may not be evident. The formula for a long life blossoming with good health is healthy diet and a regular exercise regime.

ॐ

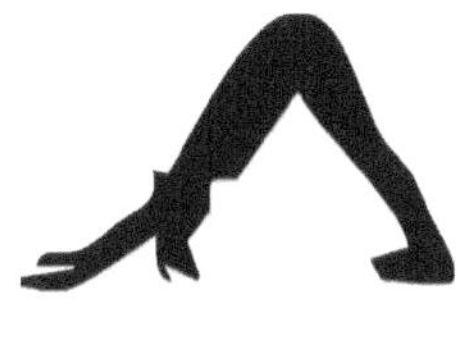

2

CHOLESTEROL
&
YOUR HEART

YOUR HEART NEEDS LOW CHOLESTEROL

Having lower cholesterol levels is very important and by now we all know this. Age is not a factor when it comes to cholesterol as we can all have a problem here. It is also a fact that you can increase your chances of having a heart attack or stroke if your cholesterol is high. We all need to understand a few of the key concepts and terms first.

Cholesterol is basically just a fat-like substance that is found throughout the body. The next thing is to know how it gets there. This is easy, you get your cholesterol through the body itself or in the foods you eat and put into it. You need to know that too much of it, however, is not healthy for the body. When your cholesterol is too high you will end up with clogged arteries which may block the heart and actually threaten to end your life. Most of us have bad cholesterol because we all love fatty foods.

There are two kinds of cholesterol that we have, which may be confusing at first. High density lipoprotein is one of them, and it is commonly known as HDL which actually needs to be high as it protects the heart from bad cholesterol. The other is low density lipoproteins, or LDL, sometimes called bad cholesterol because it can clog arteries and kill us. We have both kinds of cholesterol in our bodies and we need both. The balance between them is what gives us general good health.

Lowering your Cholesterol
For those people who would prefer not to take prescription drugs

for lowering their cholesterol, there is a more natural way. The alternative to using drugs is natural cholesterol reducers which are found in many whole foods. Most of us prefer to take natural remedies such as herbs etc. and research shows their effectiveness in getting rid of the symptoms or in reducing your chances of having heart disease.

Natural cholesterol reducers are substances that help to lower cholesterol without having to have people tamper with it first. This means that they were not created with the use of chemicals or pesticides. Garlic is considered a natural reducer because it acts as an inhibitor. Fish oils with their omega-3-fatty acids, are also known to reduce heart disease by at least 40%.

There is another factor that you need to consider. For example, did you know that Cholesterol's sister problem, beta-sitosterol, can very effectively cut blood serum cholesterol with practically no changes at all made in your diet or exercise regimens? The spice Curcumin (an extract of a curry spice turmeric), lowers cholesterol naturally. However, golgul gum resin, which is from the Myrrh tree, reduces high cholesterol levels as well as helping you with weight problems. These are just some natural spices that you can add to your diet.

80CR

CHOLESTEROL & YOUR HEART

Having lower cholesterol levels is very important to our overall health, no matter how old we are. This is especially true if we want to avoid a heart attack or stroke. We all need to understand a few of the key concepts and terms first: cholesterol, HDL, LDL, lipoproteins, serum cholesterol, dietary cholesterol, saturated fats, atherosclerosis, and coronary artery disease.

Cholesterol is basically just a fat-like substance that is found all through the body. Basically it gets there in one of two ways, either from the body itself or in the foods we eat. It is a very common and is an important worker bee in the body's honeycomb. Too much of it, however, is not healthy for the body and can clog our arteries, block our hearts, and actually threaten to end our lives. More often than not , we need to lower cholesterol in our bodies.

There are two kinds of cholesterol that we have, which may be confusing at first. High density lipoprotein is one of them, and it is commonly known as HDL, sometimes it is also called good cholesterol because it can protect the heart. Low density lipoproteins, which are commonly known as LDL, sometimes called bad cholesterol because it can clog arteries and kill us, is the other. We have both kinds of cholesterol in our bodies and we them need both. The balance between them is critical to our body. It is what helps determine whether a heart is healthy or in need of correction.

৪৩

CHOLESTEROL & HEART DISEASE

The link between cholesterol and heart disease has been established in numerous studies. Specifically, the higher the cholesterol, the greater the risk is of getting heart disease. It is really that simple. High cholesterol is common for most people. However, the good news is that we can do something about it. We all want lower cholesterol. The hard thing though is that most of us have a hard time controlling it. High cholesterol level in the blood can not only lead to heart attacks but also several weight problems.

Though cholesterol holds a thoroughly 'bad guy' image, surprisingly it serves many vital functions for healthy living. Experts today are divided into two camps: one holds cholesterol to be the sole villain while the other contradicts them saying it is not the only dominant reason for heart diseases.

Coronary heart disease or CHD, is the medical term for heart attacks. Studies have shown that having a higher level of cholesterol increases the risk of suffering CHD, while people with low cholesterol levels are less likely to have it. Hence, lowering the bad cholesterol in your blood stream seems to be a drastic solution to coronary heart diseases.

Recently, a study was conducted where statins, that are the drugs to lower the total cholesterol level, were given to some patients. This reduced their risks of suffering a heart attack phenomenally, undermining the need of undergoing bypass surgery, and of course negated risk of death from CHD-related causes.

Besides high cholesterol in the blood stream, there are some other risk factors that increase the risk of developing a heart disease. While some of them can be changed, others are undeniably here to stay. The fact remains that the more conditions you meet, the higher the risk of experiencing heart disease.

Here are the risk factors that you must know about but you cannot really help yourself in these cases:

Age
The chances of suffering CHD increase with age. For males it is 45 years and older; for females it is 55 years and older.

Genetics
In case heart troubles persist in your family history, it can be a case for you as well.

Take some time to review the factors given below thoroughly and work towards the changes as soon as possible and these are quite controllable if concentrated on in time:

High level bad cholesterol in the blood.
Lower levels of the good cholesterol in your blood.
Your history of smoking.
High Blood Pressure owing to the genetic predisposition or some family history regarding high blood pressures.
History of Diabetes and if this has some family history.
No exercise – living quite a sedentary lifestyle.
Obesity or overweight.

Some experts disagree with the fact that only high cholesterol level adds to the risk of CHD, and they rather put the blame on animal fats.

Another line of thought expounds that weight, stress and physical activity influence the level of cholesterol in our blood. While each may not be dangerous in themselves, they certainly combine in our lifestyle to deliver a lethal dose.

ଈୠ

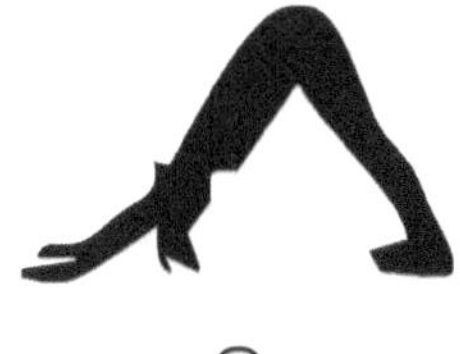

3

LEARNING TO LOWER CHOLESTEROL

LOWERING CHOLESTEROL

Most of us are at some risk for heart disease. All of us are better off if we work on lowering high cholesterol. We know that diet and exercise help as well. We know that medications are sometimes needed, and when they are, that they are most effective when combined with a healthy diet.

The cholesterol that is actually being lowered when we talk of lowering high cholesterol is LDL. It is the cholesterol that outnumbers the other cholesterol (HDL) by about 3 to 1. We are not lowering our cholesterol simply because there is more of it, even though we are trying to raise HDL because there never seems to be quite enough of it! We lower our LDL levels because of what it has a tendency to do once it has done what is required of it by our bodies – which is to help with digestion, protect the nervous system, and build cell walls. What it does and we need to stop, is build-up of blockage in our arteries.

What Helps?
Medications, of course, can be taken to chemically lower high cholesterol in the circulatory system, and it can even inhibit their being produced in the liver all together. There are synthetic and natural/herbal medications that you can use, but discussing them is a separate subject see later in the book). Dietary adjustments are particularly effective in reducing foods that which are building blocks of LDL in the liver, and those that are directly absorbed into the bloodstream.

The problem foods that do not help when you are working toward lowering high cholesterol, include such things as animal products that are high in saturated fats and processed foods and oils. Physical exercise is effective for the most part because it entails burning as energy, the molecules that otherwise accumulate in the body and bloodstream as fat, and result in overloading the vital organs, the heart being the major one.

As you will observe for yourself, when it comes to actually doing something about your cholesterol levels, a balanced diet, combined with a good fitness regimen, is your best bet. You have to be both active and eat right to maintain the right balance. You can look to the pyramid charts in the book as a means of being sure that your eating habits are balanced. Supplements of vitamins will not be able to compensate for your poor eating. You have to eat whole foods for any of this to be effective, and you must lay off heavy, fatty foods and junk food to keep your cholesterol balanced.

ॐं

LOWERING CHOLESTEROL
4 Sure-Shot Means

The human body has a complicated system that controls all aspects of life in its own peculiar way and in order to live healthy lives, we must keep all these systems intact and in control. There are several substances produced in the body that circulate in the bloodstream, with good or bad effects. For instance, insulin. It is secreted from the pancreas in response to increasing amounts of sugar that are released from the food we eat. Now the cells absorb this insulin, thereby releasing calories and energy to survive.

Another such naturally produced element is cholesterol, a major cause of heart disease. High cholesterol level in the blood not only leads to heart attacks but also causes several weight problems. Cholesterol is a waxy, fat-like substance made naturally in the liver. Though cholesterol holds a thoroughly 'bad guy' image, it surprisingly serves many vital functions for healthy living. Basically, cholesterol is of two types:
- Low Density Lipoprotein or LDL
- High-Density Lipoprotein or HDL

Low Density Lipoprotein or LDL
- This is the actual bad guy. It is this type of cholesterol that clogs blood vessels leading to increased risks of heart attack and other heart diseases.
- Researchers have now proved that a diet comprising of highly saturated fats increases the level of LDL cholesterol in the body.

High-Density Lipoprotein or HDL
- This is 'the good guy' or to be more specific, the favorable

type of cholesterol. It clears 'the bag guy', that is the LDL cholesterol from our bloodstream, thereby reducing the risk of all heart ailments.
- Research has shown that a diet rich in fruit and vegetables along with average levels of omega-3 from fish oil, greatly helps raise HDL cholesterol levels.

When you get a blood test done to check the cholesterol level in the bloodstream, the report will have a breakdown of LDL and HDL. These figures are not as important for doctors as the other two figures: total cholesterol and triglyceride level. You will only be given a clean bill of health if these readings remain within a certain range, which are:
- Total Cholesterol: equal to or less than 200mg/dl.
- Triglyceride Level: equal to or less than 150mg/dl.

On a positive note, with four simple ways one can work on gradually reducing the cholesterol levels of the body. These are?

1. Change your Diet
Focus less on the high saturated fats like red meat and dairy products. Replace them with fruits, fish, oatmeal, nuts and vegetables.

Studies have proved that consuming oatmeal regularly for two weeks reduces LDL cholesterol and triglycerides considerably. Imagine its impact if you continue to do that for over a month or so?

2. Exercise
Exercising is the healthiest of all resorts against cholesterol and the most effective in the long run. Exercising increases your heart rate and improves the metabolism of the body allowing improved expulsion of harmful oils which are detrimental to health. What type of exercises you must do, completely depends on various factors including age, gender and weight, along with your medical history.

Those who are new to a regular exercise regimen should first consult their physicians and check out what is safe for them and what is not. Those already suffering from heart trouble may not be advised any rigorous exercise but simpler alternates like stretching, weight-lifting, walking, etc. Should our physician allow you to participate in some high impact exercise, try swimming, running, bicycling, aerobics, etc. Ask your doctor to sketch your fitness plan in detail and stick to the same with the guidance of a professional fitness trainer. As a good patient and a responsible individual, following the plan is in your hands. Exercising is better than all other remedies as it has few side-effects other than healthy ones!

3. Vitamins Supplements and Drugs

While CHD does not react instantly, it gradually develops as a person ages and with sustained high levels of cholesterol. In order to live a healthy and long life it is a must for you to lower the cholesterol levels as early as possible. Here are some specialized medications and substitutes to fight back rising cholesterol levels. Studies show that their regular in take can lower the cholesterol level from 15-30%.

- Bile acid resins
- Ezetimibe
- Fibric acid
- Niacin
- Statins

However, these do have many side-effects so do not try to medicate yourself. Consult your doctor before taking any of them. Remember there are a numbers of brands selling these drugs that you can choose from and it is for your doctor to decide which one would be the best option for you.

4. Regular Check-Ups

Prevention is simply the best cure to any disease. Hence, remember to follow through on your regular check-ups with the doctor. That little expenditure will save you the large hospital bill that could come up in future.

॰॥

LOWERING CHOLESTEROL THE NATURAL WAY

For those people who prefer not to take prescription drugs to lower cholesterol, there are alternatives – natural cholesterol reducers. Many people prefer them to taking medication as they are believed to be safer. An increasing number of studies are being conducted on the medicinal value of naturally occurring substances such as herbs, flowers and plants. Results show their effectiveness in alleviating symptoms and reducing chances of heart disease. The choice is up to the individual.

What Exactly Are Natural Cholesterol Reducers?

Natural cholesterol reducers are regularly seen as substances occurring without human intervention. This effectively means they were not created with the use of chemicals or pesticides. A large number of them have been the subject of recent studies, and have been proven effective as natural cholesterol reducers. Garlic is on the list as a significant inhibitor to the development of arteriosclerosis and an aid in disabling the recurrence of heart attacks. Fish oils possess their omega-3-fatty acids and are commonly known to reduce heart disease occurrences by as much as 45 percent.

Cholesterol's close relative, called beta-sitosterol, can effectively cut blood serum cholesterol with practically no changes made in your diet or exercise regimen. Curcumin, which is the extract of a curry spice (turmeric), lowers cholesterol as well as helping in other areas of general health. However, if we move a bit farther on into the exotic spices, we learn that golgul gum resin that comes from the myrrh tree, reduces high cholesterol levels as well helping with with weight problems.

A specific sugarcane wax derivative called policosanol, prevents LDL from oxidizing in the bloodstream. Psyllium, which is the fibre of a plant that is native to India and Iran, also lowers LDL levels. It is important to note that Ogul Gum Resin, Garlic, Curcumin, and Policosanol only have limited effectiveness because they only last for about six months. This is because they are exogenic. So it is a good idea to look for endogenic supplements such as Beta Sitosterol, Beta Glucan, Chromax and soy isoflavones, to assist you in your efforts.

How You Should Use Natural Cholesterol Reducers

Any medication that you choose to take should be used based on living a healthy lifestyle which includes exercise and diet control and better overall daily habits that are conducive to your good health. It does not cost much to live a healthier lifestyle if only one tries. This just proves that lowering the cholesterol can be done which is much better than ending up in the hospital with complications. This means that you are required to undertake some regular physical exercise, maintain a moderate body weight and always insist on a balanced diet as part of your normal lifestyle. Lifestyle is the greatest contributor to health. This is true for cholesterol levels and particularly for LDL, because this is the cholesterol that is driven so strongly by your diet. HDL is not an exception to this rule either, simply that it is influenced by other factors as well. Medications alone are usually not enough to ensure long-term health.

Studies have shown that the number of people who are obese or overweight has gone up dramatically through the years. This is attributed to the type of food being served in schools and fast food joints as well the lack of physical activity as the person grows older. The problem goes farther because this means that many more people will suffer from high blood pressure, heart disease and strokes in the future. The good news is that this can be prevented before it is too late.

The natural way to lower cholesterol is by making some lifestyle changes and exercising regularly. This will help lose weight, which is directly related to the cholesterol levels in the human body.

When people think of dieting, many think this means saying

goodbye to some of life's more delicious foods, but it is not so. A person has to limit the consumption of these and add new things that are healthier. This will require eating foods that are high in fibre and low in saturated fats. A few examples of these are artichokes, corn, fish, garlic, legumes, mushrooms, nut, olive oil, soy milk and whole grains. One should not forget to have some fruits and vegetables regularly since these are rich in sterols that are known to keep cholesterol levels down. All of these products are affordable and easily available.

Apart from a healthy diet, one must take the necessary precautions when consuming liquids. This means moderate drinking of a glass of red wine, reducing the consumption of beer, drinking fresh juices, non-fat milk and water. One is strongly encouraged to drink lots of water. Unsweetened tea is also safe to drink. It may taste different so mixing a sachet of Equal or NutraSweet can add some flavoring. Apple juice for example, has been known to reduce cholesterol levels by up to 50% when taken regularly. Other fruits can also do the same, so chopping up some fresh fruit and putting it into a blender can help you preserve this aid to good health in bottled form.

Changing the way food is cooked is also another way to reduce cholesterol naturally. Instead of frying, one can try steaming, boiling or the quick way – using the microwave. There was a time that doctors encourage children and adults to drink milk. Though this can help strengthen the bones as one ages, this too is has certain ingredients that are not safe. This should be changed for soy or non-fat milk that may taste a little different but is much healthier.

Cholesterol is something that is produced in the body and is also ingested with food. The only way to make sure the levels in the blood do not exceed the limit, is to have regular check-ups and watch the food that is being served in restaurants you patronise.

The next step to lowering cholesterol levels naturally is through exercise. This can be achieved in many ways such as brisk walking, jogging or running around the neighborhood. Those who want to be looked after by a personal trainer can check out the gym since there are professionals that can create a program to achieve the desired results. This will be a combination of cardio-vascular exercises as well as weight-lifting to burn calories and lower cholesterol levels. Studies have shown that getting those muscles to work is much better and safer than taking prescription drugs that are known to have certain side effects when it is taken. The same goes for the use of food supplements since the human body needs exercise to keep in functioning.

There is another way to reduce cholesterol levels but is only used as a last resort if the other two do not work. One is required to use medication to make it happen. There are many products available and studies have shown they can drop cholesterol levels by as much as 15% to 30%. One should be aware though that these drugs have certain side-effects so it is best to consult a doctor first to make sure it is safe to use.

Cholesterol is just one of the substances that the body makes on its own. Unfortunately, eating food that is high in oil and saturated fats creates an imbalance. If precautions are not taken, the chances of a heart attack and other cardiovascular diseases get higher as the person ages. Cholesterol is classified into two. The first is called LDL or low-density lipoprotein. This is better known as bad cholesterol and having too much of it can cause problems in the health of an individual. It is a good thing that the body can counter this with HDL or high-density lipoprotein, which is called good cholesterol. There must a balance between the two so that the heart, blood circulation and all the other systems are working as they should.

The only way for the patient to know the cholesterol levels in the body is through a blood test. Those who fall within 4.4 to 7.1, have a small chance of experiencing a heart attack. Any figure above that is bad and anything below means the risks are much lower.

₧ℂℛ

NATURAL WAYS OF REDUCING CHOLESTEROL
Best Alternatives

The key cause of heart diseases, as the doctors suggest, is cholesterol. High cholesterol level in the blood can not only lead to heart attacks but also several weight problems. In fact, it has now become the Number 1 cause of death in all developed countries. Coronary heart disease or the CHD is the medical term for heart attacks. Lowering the bad cholesterol in your bloodstream seems to be the effective solution to coronary heart diseases.

CHD does not happen instantly, it gradually develops with a person's age and through sustained high cholesterol. In order to live a healthy and long life it is essential to lower the cholesterol levels as early as possible. Though unhealthy eating habits are the key to growing cholesterol ailments, it is not the only one. The other reasons for the same are:

- **Age**: the chances of suffering CHD increases with age. For males it is 45 years and older; for females it is 55 years and older.
- **Genetics**: in case heart troubles persist in your family history, it can be a strong indicator in your case as well.

Take some time to review the factors in the list below and work towards the changes as soon as possible. These are quite controllable if concentrated on in time.
- High level of bad cholesterol in the blood.
- Low levels of the good cholesterol in your blood.
- Your history of smoking.

- High Blood Pressure owing to genetic predisposition.
- History of Diabetes and if this has some family history.
- No exercise – living a sedentary lifestyle.
- Obesity or overweight.

Consult your physician if you suffering with high blood cholesterol and take his words seriously in order to live a healthy life. There are several natural ways to reduce and control the cholesterol in our bodies.

Diet
A low cholesterol diet primarily includes:
- Grains, mainly whole grain products and cereals.
- Fish rich in Omega3, like Salmon and Tuna.
- Fruits and leafy vegetables.
- Nuts.
- Fresh juices.

The following tips are useful to remember.
- Visit your physician prior to initializing any low cholesterol diet. This will help you gauge the improvements and changes in your health.
- Replace the saturated fats with polyunsaturated fats in chicken, meat and whole milk products.
- Try to avoid pastas, sugar, sugar-coated foods and bakery products that contain refined carbohydrates.
- While eating out, opt for boiled, steamed or salad food.

Vitamin Supplements & Medication
Here are some of the specialized medications and substitutes used to fight back rising cholesterol levels instantly:
- **Statins**: these are specialized medications aimed at lowering cholesterol levels. Such medications are grouped into different classes. The most common ones available in the market are HMG-CoA Inhibitors, or statins. Statins reduce the cholesterol in our body by blocking the enzyme HMG-CoA. Formation of this enzyme is one of the important functions in the steps involved in the conversion of fats into cholesterol. These are the most effective drugs for lowering cholesterol. Hence, they have been of great help to people

who require urgent and drastic reduction in their
cholesterol levels.

- **Bile Acid Sequestrants**: the human liver produces a special
bile and these cholesterol lowering drugs bind with the bile.
Bile is a substance that aids our digestive system to absorb
fats. Bile acid sequestrant prevents cholesterol from forming
by prevents the bile acid from digesting the fats.
- **Vitamin B3 /Niacin:** Vitamin B3 or Niacin, is the most
common cholesterol lowering vitamin. It is one among the
8 water-soluble B vitamins. It helps the body in the
conversion of carbohydrates into glucose which provides
energy. B vitamins are also important in breaking down body
fats, as well as proteins and acids, which aid in making the
nervous system, eyes, skin, mouth, hair and liver healthy.
Niacin is also helpful in getting rid of toxic and harmful
chemicals from the body.
Niacin increases the effect of the other cholesterol reducing
drugs, but only if taken in very high doses. This is not very
advisable as taking large amounts of Vitamin B can lead to
flushing of the skin which happens due to the dilation of
blood vessels. Other side-effects of excessive intake of
Vitamin B3 are headaches, itching, muscle cramps and nausea.
Lecithin are among the other substances and vitamins that
lower body cholesterol. It allows cholesterol and fats to
disperse from the body and prevents fatty build-up in the arteries.
- **Vitamins C and E:** Vitamins C & E prevent LDL cholesterol
from damage, hence saving people from heart disease.
While LDL cholesterol is also known to be the bad guy, most
cardiologists believe that only damaged LDL cholesterol
contributes to the rising risk of heart diseases.

It would nevertheless be worth spending the time to consult
your doctor on ways to reduce cholesterol through a healthy lifestyle
and natural means.

₨₭

LOWERING THE INSTANT RISE IN BAD CHOLESTEROL LEVELS

Studies show that the genes we inherit are closely related to the rise of cholesterol levels. This rise is also due to several other factors like:

- Unhealthy lifestyle.
- Unhealthy eating habits: saturated fat and high calorie intake.
- Lack of exercise.
- Excessive drinking.
- Menopausal stage in women, when estrogen begins to diminish.
- Age factor: senior citizens often suffer from this condition.

Low Density Lipoprotein or LDL

- It is the actual bad guy. It is this type of cholesterol that clogs blood vessels leading to increased risks of heart attack and other heart diseases.
- Researchers have now proved that a diet comprising of highly saturated fats increases the level of LDL cholesterol in the body.

High-Density Lipoprotein or HDL

- This is the good guy or to be more specific, the favorable type of cholesterol. It clears 'the bag guy' that is LDL cholesterol from our bloodstream, thereby reducing the risk of all heart ailments.
- Researchers have shown that a diet rich in fruit and vegetables along with average levels of omega-3 from fish oil, greatly helps raise HDL cholesterol levels.

In the absence of any remedial measures, the rising levels of LDL cholesterol can lead to heart ailments, high blood pressure, etc. Here are some ways to lower your cholesterol levels instantly.

- Most people believe that exercising regularly, eating the right diet without saturated animal fats, diary and lard, is the final solution to treating the high cholesterol levels. But, going by these foods' lipid sources, it shows that they cannot create an instant suspension of the unwanted elements in the body. They have no side-effects on various cardiovascular diseases and disorders in the artheroma degeneration related to arterial walls.

- To instantly decrease the rising cholesterol level in blood, statins are considered quite effective. Crestor (rosuvastatin calcium): this medication puts a halt on very high bad cholesterol levels. It reduces it by 52% with a 10mg dosage, as compared to a 7 mg placebo. Crestor increases HDL cholesterol (the good cholesterol), by 14%, versus 3% up HDL cholesterol of the placebo. It works both ways, reducing LDL cholesterol and increasing HDL cholesterol. So it is a really significant pro-life saving drug.

You must inform your licensed physician regarding the factors listed below in order to undergo effective treatment.
- Liver and kidney problems.
- Pregnancy.
- Excessive or normal drinking – the liver is highly affected by alcohol.
- Family history of high cholesterol cases.
- Problems like diabetes and hypothyroidism.
- Any recent incidents of heart and/or hypertension attack.
- Other disease that do not pertain to high cholesterol.
- Chinese and/or Japanese ancestry.
- Consumption of over-the-counter medicines that are antacids.
- All your other prescriptions.

The side-effects of Crestor are :
- Constipation.
- Muscle aches.

- Abdominal pain.
- Weakness.
- Nausea.

Though these are all quite mild symptoms and all go away in due course, patients in such cases must take care that they minimize their intake of fatty unsaturated substances. In this regard here are some important points.

- Cooking in olive oil is the best for such patients as it reduces the fatty unsaturated acids to a great extent.
- A report made by Dr. P. Rethinam & Mohartuyo, quoted in the *Jakarta Post* on 18 June 2003, confirms that coconut oil is the best vegetable oil to control bad cholesterol in the body, among all other vegetable oils such as corn, sunflower, soy, rapeseed, cottonseed and palm kernel.

ഈ⊗

BAD CHOLESTEROL
WHAT IT IS & HOW DOES IT WORK?

Basically, cholesterol is of two types:
- Low Density Lipoprotein or LDL
- High-Density Lipoprotein or HDL

Low Density Lipoprotein or LDL is the bad guy. It is this type of cholesterol that clogs the blood vessels leading to increased risks of heart attack and other heart diseases. Researchers have now proved that diet comprising of highly saturated fats increases the level of LDL cholesterol in the body.

Understanding some medical terms regarding cholesterol is important. Atheroma is caused by bad cholesterol or LDL. It is a plaque in the arteries – or in a layman's language, fat streaks. If not monitored, the accumulation of macrophage white blood cells can even happen to a 10 year-old child.

In such cases, the early but quiet and slow symptoms start developing in the child at the tender age of 5. As the child grows, the veins get choked with accumulations. Often, the exact symptoms show up only after the on-set of a heart attack or stroke. Unfortunately, it comes to the surface when it is already late. This type of stroke often acts as a silent killer that may cause death or lifetime disability.

It is difficult to imagine how high levels of bad cholesterol can lead to serious consequences for the body. Though some people appear to be healthy on the surface, their ailment only shows up with lab tests – the results of which often come as a surprise or shock.

The hidden facts behind this drastic rise of bad cholesterol in the body is simple enough – high intake of saturated fats in the diet. It takes just a minute to read through the labels or guides of processed foods. They all clearly mention the amount of cholesterol that food contains.

In order to understand the functioning of cholesterol in the body, we must first understand how it gets metabolized in the body.

Cholesterol does not come from food alone. Diet is just one of the factors and there are several other mechanisms attached to this process. Good cholesterol supports the biochemical functioning of the body like producing bile and regulating fat soluble vitamins like K, A, E, and D.

Cholesterol also makes a great impact on our body's synthesis of hormones. Right after the cholesterol is utilized in the body, it excretes in the form of excess lipids into the gall bladder and liver as crystal particles. Cholesterol is not soluble in water. Hence, it circulates in the body over and over again until it gets converted into bad cholesterol or low density lipoproteins. The bad cholesterol comes in a number of small sizes and is usually trapped in our veins as accumulated clogs.

In healthy individuals, the metabolism is smooth whereby bad cholesterol minimizes. The key to lowering high cholesterol is simply watching over your diet and having no genetic weaknesses. Avoid foods where cholesterol or fatty oils are prevalent in excess like animal meats and fats, especially beef and pork.

Try and discipline your life and you could work better on your less cholesterol diet!

ॐकर

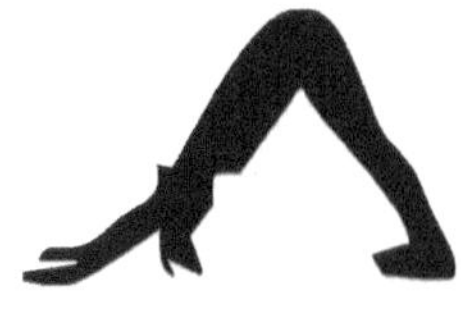

4

FOOD & CHOLESTEROL

FOOD FOR PEOPLE WITH HIGH CHOLESTEROL

Bad cholesterol sticks to the body and refuses to let go. For those affected, efforts to lower cholesterol levels can prove futile and very frustrating. If only water could flush out all the bad cholesterol from the body! Bad cholesterol clogs the veins. Even though they have a tiny diameter, this can cause a hindrance to the smooth flow of blood which can even be fatal.

It is a common misconception that all cholesterol is bad for heath. Good cholesterol is important for all the vital processes of the human body. The bad cholesterol is the one that clogs arteries. However it takes many years of unchecked dietary habits to gradually build up to the level when cholesterol can be fatal.

Cholesterol usually affects obese or overweight people. The factors that adversely affect people are drugs, bad diet and hereditary traits. As a result, cholesterol in people with normal weight is comparatively rarer, but not unheard of.

There is not much information available about prevention of cholesterol. Most of the available literature talks about reduction of cholesterol levels after a person has been diagnosed clinically. Maintaining a healthy lifestyle is the most effective method of preventing various health disorders to begin with. Although this is talked about all the time, carefully watching over your food consumption is often overlooked but remains the most practical way of preventing bad health and obesity.

Various food groups help in lowering of cholesterol levels. Such foodstuffs contain antioxidants that prevent the increase of bad cholesterol levels in the body. These include:

FIBERS including OATMEAL
This is a fibre of high nutritional content with the capability of reducing cholesterol. Many studies were conducted on this in the 1980's, right up until 1989. However, it lost its popularity temporarily till 1997, when it was revived again by the Food and Drug Administration after it was declared that combined with a good diet that is low in fat, it can prevent various heart diseases.

Other fibrous foods include legumes, rice, brewer's yeast, bran, wheat, breads, beans and various other cereals that help in increasing the levels of good cholesterol in the body.

FRUITS & VEGETABLES
These are full of vitamins and antioxidants and are found at the top of the food pyramid. It is necessary that we eat lots of these natural foods rather than processed foods. They cleanse the body and are healthy as they do not contain any fats. Citrus fruits that contain vitamin C should be particularly favoured. The best medicine to combat free-radical elements that cause various diseases is cucumber, as it is rich in the anti-oxidant vitamin E.

FISH
Fish with white meat and Tuna, are also a part of healthy diets as they contain smaller amounts of unsaturated fats.

LEAN MEATS
Extra lean beef, liver, turkey and chicken without skin, are all fat-free and rich in proteins. Therefore, they are integral to a healthy diet.

YOUGRT
It helps in the digestion of food by regulating stomach acids. Hence it aids the reduction of cholesterol levels and is also low in fat.

෨෧

FOOD TO LOWER CHOLESTEROL

'We are what we eat.' How true! The food we eat determines the cholesterol levels of our body. High cholesterol levels can cause heart diseases and high blood pressure as age progresses and lead to paralysis or death. Unless several important changes are made in diet, high cholesterol levels can steal lives. Almost all of the most popular foods stuffs contain large quantities of LDC, known more popularly as 'bad cholesterol'. By substituting these with HDL, widely known as 'good cholesterol', we can have a much healthier life. Given below are some of the best ways to do this.

Breakfast is the most important meal of the day. Bread should be avoided and be replaced by oatmeal. Doing this ensures that in just two weeks the cholesterol levels in the body will be reduced by almost 20%. Making this a habit will greatly reduce the cholesterol levels of the body.

If breakfast cannot contain oatmeal, fruit such as apples should be had. Having two apples or twelve ounces of good apple juice a day, can lower the chance of various diseases of the heart by almost 50%. Apples can be had as dessert or a snack or even after a light meal.

Making vegetables a part of lunch and dinner is the most effective way to ensure a healthy diet. Also red meat should be replaced with fish or poultry. These food stuffs are healthier as they do not contain saturated fats.

People who love cooking can add ingredients such as garlic to their food. Garlic has the property of declogging arteries thereby reducing the chances of getting heart diseases.

Beans are good for health. A helping of beans twice or thrice a week can greatly reduce the risk of bad cholesterol as they contain fibres that are soluble and can help in fighting bad cholesterol. Onions are not always popular but having just half an onion per day greatly reduces LDC and increases HDC in the body.

There is a popular misconception that all fats are bad for health. This is not entirely correct. There are different kinds of fats. Some are bad for the health while others like omega 3 fatty acids and unsaturated fats are considered to be healthy.

The way food is prepared greatly affects the cholesterol levels of the body. Cooking oils contain monosaturated and polysaturated fats which are highly effective in lowering cholesterol levels in the body. Hence food should be cooked using these oils. While shopping, the ingredients of the item should be properly read from the label in order to ensure that it is healthy.

People who are overweight and flabby are the ones who are most likely to suffer from various diseases caused by high levels of bad cholesterol. If making a personalized dietary plan is difficult, then a dietitian should be consulted to customize one. This then has to be followed religiously.

ജ്ഞ

FOODS TO AVOID TO LOWER CHOLESTEROL

Basically people just love to eat. Any free time they get they do not miss out on catching up on a meal. The meal we are talking about here is not one of the three basic meals one has during the course of the day, but one of the inter-meal cravings one indulges in. In other words, snack breaks. Rare does one pay attention to what exactly the cholesterol content in the food we are consuming is. The ultimate pleasure lies only in savouring the taste. These snacks, often picked up from fast food centres, are extremely unhealthy and have a high cholesterol content ,which has even encouraged McDonalds to mention the calorie content in every product.

The alarming growth in the number of obese and overweight people is something to take note of. The obvious implications of this are the number of people who are now prone to heart diseases and heart attacks. Many suggestions have been made to try to curb this growing trend. They include annually check-ups and making changes to one's daily habits and lifestyle. The only way to reduce the cholesterol intake is to be conscious about your diet. Reduce the amount going into your system.

What kind of food has very high in cholesterol content? What food must you avoid? Here is a simple guide.

- First and foremost if you are a voracious red meat eater, you must definitely cut down on the steak, bacon and ham. They are extremely high in fat content.
- Foregoing it at one instant will be hard for an individual,

hence the age old technique of divide and conquer must be adopted. One can start by gradually decreasing the amount of such food content.

- The oil and constituent ingredients used to cook fried foods like burgers and French fries are a store house of cholesterol and fat. This list also includes frozen meals which have been pre-packaged.
- Dairy and Poultry products like eggs, milk and chicken should be minimized in one's diet. To ensure that the body gets sufficient amounts of calcium, one can include non-fat milk and yogurt in the diet.
- Junk food is not as much of a threat when we are children as in adulthood. Eventually as one grows older, the dietary necessities must be taken into consideration.

Above we have mentioned the food items one must avoid. Apart from fat and cholesterol these may also be considered vital elements of a diet. Hence, we look into substitutes for these food items.

- Products such as fruits, soy, whole wheat grain and vegetables must be taken aplenty. These products have omega 3 acids which reduce the cholesterol content in the human body apart from delivering the essential vitamins and minerals required.
- One must adopt the motto 'eat less and live long' and make sure the diet one consumes must be within the limit of 30 percent cholesterol.

For special and specific needs, one should visit a dietician for further guidance who will set up a daily dietary pattern with variations.

శుభం

FOLLOWING A LOW CHOLESTEROL PLAN

It is a fact that higher cholesterol levels lead to a range of diseases. The amount of cholesterol in the human body can be reduced by adopting various techniques. If we notice the food patterns adopted by a majority of people, we notice the tendency to consume more food which is high in LDL which is the bad cholesterol.

Sedentary lifestyle is a big no-no and it is essential to incorporate a regular exercise regime in one's daily routine. Bad habits like smoking and drinking are major contributors to the increasing cholesterol levels. On a long-term basis this paves the way for various heart diseases. In much of the Western world, heart diseases are considered prime killers. People have to be educated that reducing the amount of LDL cholesterol,can significantly reduce the risk of heart attacks.

The earlier one puts these changes into practice the better and there will be lesser probability of one suffering from heart disease.

A healthy lifestyle includes
- a balanced diet consisting of all the essential vitamins, minerals, proteins, carbohydrates and fiber;
- drinking sufficient amounts of water;
- developing a regular exercise regime.

If one wishes to develop a formula for a dietary plan which will help reduce the amount of cholesterol, one should have a precise idea in mind of what one will be doing. One must be mentally prepared. If one is mentally prepared; focused on the goals and determined about following the low cholesterol diet, there is higher probability of success and that one will adhere to it with more heart and soul for a longer period.

Prior to jumping onto a strict diet regime to ensure lower cholesterol levels, one should do some research on what food types are recommended and which are not and why. The main thought process while starting a low cholesterol diet plan is to reduce the consumption of saturated fats, calories and cholesterol. This effort not only helps in the lowering cholesterol levels but also plays a role in weight reduction which is an extra bonus!

As mentioned earlier the primary food items to be consumed to ensure best results are fruits and vegetables. These not only have vitamins, but are also high in fibre content. One can think of fiber as something like a sponge ball which absorbs all the cholesterol and helps dispose of it. Fruits like pears, apples and oranges have high fibre content as do carrots. Oats are highly recommended too.

ဆာ၏

THE BEST LOW CHOLESTEROL DIET PLAN

Having the perfect balanced diet is one of the keys to maintaining cholesterol levels at the lower end. A long proven fact is that cholesterol levels and the risk of developing coronary heart diseases, is directly proportional to each other. This is potentially very dangerous.

Taking medicines may reduce the level of cholesterol in the body but the healthier option is definitely to opt for a more cholesterol free diet. Consumption of products like soy products, green, leafy vegetables and other special low cholesterol food products, are effective options. Studies have also shown that one can lower cholesterol levels by about one third within a month by sticking to a vegetarian diet.

Vegetables like red pepper and broccoli (healthy portions mind you), soy products such as soy sausages and soymilk, serving of oats , bran, cereal and whole wheat bread, and plenty of fresh fruits and certain nuts, constitute an effective low cholesterol diet. The products mentioned above, especially nuts and fibre-rich products like barley, oats and soy protein, can reduce cholesterol levels by as much as seventy percent.

A diet low in cholesterol content makes it mandatory for one to reduce the intake of fatty substances by around 25 to 30 percent and saturated fats by 70%. Consumption of non-hydrogenated (unprocessed) fats, in comparison to the hydrogenated variety, is considered to be one of the ideal components for reducing the risk of coronary heart ailments. By increasing the intake of fish oil, omega-3 fats from fish or plant sources such as flaxseed, is the recommended forms of fat consumption while following a low cholesterol diet. Apart from this, one's intake of sodium should also be brought down to around 2400 milligrams per day.

One can plan one's day in the following way.
- The first meal of the day, breakfast, can consist of bran oat cereal with healthy nuts like almond or walnut, fruit salad, soymilk, whole wheat or oatmeal bread and jam.
- The next meal of the day, lunch, should consist of bean soup along with bran bread, soy nuts and end with a bowl of fruit.
- Dinner can consist of tofu, almonds, fruit and stir-fry vegetables.

If one follows this regime with heart and soul, not deviating from it, a large difference of about 29 percent drop in cholesterol level in one month can be achieved.

ଚଢ

LOWER YOUR CHOLESTEROL WITH ACCURATE DIET: 11 Easy Tips

While wrong diet is the single major cause of rising cholesterol levels in the bloodstream, experts suggest there are several other factors as well that trigger this problem. These include:

- Genetics
- Little physical activity
- Obesity
- Unhealthy lifestyle eg. excessive smoking and drinking
- Hormones
- Varying high and low cholesterol levels

Cholesterol Healthy Diet

As cholesterol is becoming a common health problem across the globe now, experts suggest that people over 20 years old should be aware of the problem and adapt their lifestyles to lower LDL cholesterol in the body before it becomes a problem.

While it may not be easy to follow the actual requisites in totality, experts say that this problem can be combated with the consumption of proper diet at least. Low cholesterol level can surely ensure less or no risk of heart ailments and for that you need a controlled and regulated diet. However, since this is a hard nut to crack, it is simpler to take the right foods knowing the effective cholesterol formulas.

11 easy tips on the perfect cholesterol free diet

1   A low cholesterol diet primarily includes the following:
- Grains – mainly whole grain products and cereals.

- Fish rich in Omega3, like Salmon and Tuna.
- Fruits and leafy vegetables.
- Nuts.
- Juices, etc.

2   Visit your physician prior to initializing any low cholesterol diet. This will help you gauge improvements and changes in your health.

3   Replace saturated fats with polyunsaturated fats in chicken, meat and whole milk products.

4   Try to avoid pastas, sugar, sugar-coated foods and bakery products as they contain refined carbohydrates which add to cholesterol levels.

5   While eating out, opt for boiled, steamed or grilled food preparations.

6   If possible, pick out lean fish, meat and skinless chicken that are baked, broiled, steamed, grilled, Poached – that is, anything but fried.

7   Focus on vegetable side dishes and fresh fruit desserts.

8   Try avoiding margarine, eggs and butter in your regular diet.

9   Use natural-based oils such as corn, vegetable, olive, etc. for cooking.

10   Add lots of garlic while cooking. It lowers the HDL cholesterol level tremendously.

11   Add plenty of high quality vitamin and mineral supplements to your diet: such as Vitamin E, which improves blood circulation; Vitamin C & Vitamin B3, that lower high cholesterol levels, etc.

ℰᴏᴄℜ

LOWER THE CHOLESTEROL LEVEL WITH A HEALTHY DIET: 8 Easy Tips

Reality shows have become popular with their natural presentation and real emotions, with no pre-written scripts like other television series. The events unfold naturally in the course of viewing and inspire you in many ways. One such show has been the American series, *The Biggest Loser*. Inspiring viewers to become healthy and fighting fit once again, the contestants on this show were an interesting bunch of overweight people, both men and women, working out thoroughly and following a strictly balanced diet. They focused their full devotion to reducing their weight. At the end of each week, 1 player was eliminated. The winner was the one who shed the most pounds in three months for a prize worth $250,000. It was also a golden second chance to live a healthy life.

The contestants were fighting for much more than money – their own life and health were the issues being tackled. Workouts are considered to be the healthiest way of reducing fats in the body. This is perhaps the fastest way of cutting down those excess deposits beneath your skin but after the workout what you require is some energy back-up. This meal, which follows right after the workout, must be a balanced diet with the right amount of proteins, carbohydrates, fats, etc. This meal repairs damaged tissues, refuels energy and lowers cholesterol.

While lowering cholesterol will not happen overnight, observing a proper diet along with exercises, helps to lose those extra pounds and considerably cut the cholesterol levels.

Here are some examples of food, which taken after a workout, will help you minimize cholesterol.

1.   Those of you who prefer having bread after working out, consider substituting regular bread with wheat bread, as certain ingredients in regular bread are rich sources of the bad cholesterol. Wheat bread is much healthier.

2.   As nuts also help a great deal in lowering cholesterol levels, try having sandwiches with low fat peanut butter.

3.   Fruits are perhaps the best way to lower cholesterol levels. Experts advise consuming the fruits whole rather than peeling off the skin or making them into juices. Studies suggest that eating fruit in its natural form keeps their natural fibers intact which in turn contributes to your health

4.   After your gym session, simply eat from a home-made packet containing some sticks of carrot or sliced tomatoes. This is also perfect food with which to push off to office directly from the gym.

5.   Returning from the work, all of us crave for some filling food. Have some chicken or fish that is baked in a microwave or simple steamed. Experts explain that fried food is full of cooking oils that shoot up cholesterol levels tremendously. So try cooking in ways other than frying.

6.   Add plenty of vegetables to your meals.

7.   Garlic and onions are quite easy to add to your regular food and these are helpful in lowering the liver's cholesterol production.

8.   The last meal of the day must end with some yogurt. This will leave you satisfied but light.

৪৩

LOWERING CHOLESTEROL WITH GOOD DIET:
An Easy-to-Follow Meal

Raj is a healthy, cautious and responsible individual who exercises twice a week and loves to try all kinds of food. He is a family man with a wife and two children. He recently underwent an annual physical examination and blood test. The results are changing his life. The reports read that LDL cholesterol or the commonly called 'bad cholesterol', was far higher in his blood than the HDL cholesterol or 'good cholesterol'. The doctor has warned Raj to adapt his lifestyle or else he could suffer high blood pressure, heart attack or stroke.

Here are the key points of advice the doctor gave Raj.
- Increase the workout to four days a week instead of two days.
- Engage in other activities that help to lower cholesterol, such as swimming or other sport.
- The right intake of food. After all, exercising makes no sense if one keeps consuming the unwanted elements and infusing them into the body. The food consumed must not supply cholesterol that one is working out to burn. So the doctor referred Raj to a dietician.

Raj had a long discussion with the dietician who explained which food can be replaced with what and what exactly he needed to cut down on. This was the diet plan the dietician gave Raj.

- The food would now contain low fats and no rich carbohydrates.

- The breakfast would comprise of the yellow portion of egg without the white.
- Morning coffee would be replaced with unsweetened tea.
- Raj could also have cereals with his children. But he will have to stick to non-fat milk.
- For lunch, something heavier can be considered. Skinless chicken with a reduced portion of steak are good options.
- Lots of vegetables and other such side dishes with lunch.
- As the new diet plan is something very different from the usual, initially it will not be easy for Raj and he will feel hungry again by late afternoon. At this time, some fruit or salad can be had – perhaps some carrot sticks or an apple. This is a much healthier option that a donut loaded with sugar.
- With the snack, while Raj usually had a Coke, now he has to shift to plain water or fresh fruit juice. Not the packaged juices which are full of sugar again.
- Before going to bed, dinner would be some fish or pasta, along with some side vegetables.
- In terms of drinks, beer is out. Raj can have the occasional glass of red wine.
- It is important point to remember that this diet plan has to be followed even at a party or eating out at a restaurant. Health diet charts have no day off, nor do risks of heart disease, high blood pressure, etc.

If Raj follows this plan strictly for a few weeks, his doctor expects a tremendous improvement in his condition in the next check up. The aim would be to lower the LDL cholesterol.

There are many alternatives to what was suggested for Raj. Do take the time to research and discuss what suits your needs. Lower your cholesterol and live healthy again!

৪৩

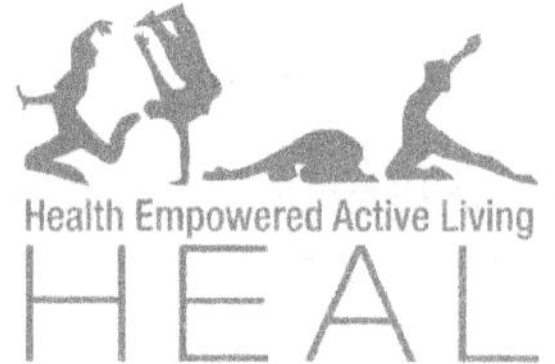
Health Empowered Active Living
HEAL

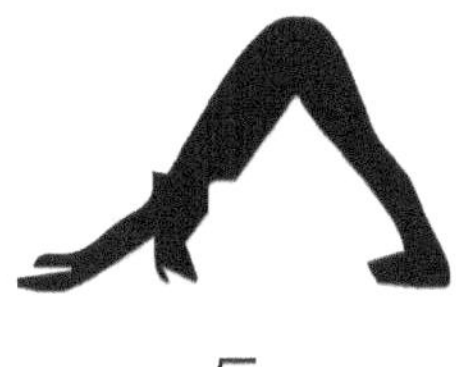

5

MEDICATIONS & CHOLESTEROL

A DRUG-FREE WAY TO LOWER CHOLESTEROL

In the recent years the number of people suffering from high cholesterol levels has increased substantially. Studies have proven that many heart diseases are caused primarily by high levels of cholesterol in the body. This results in heart attacks and strokes which can sometimes prove fatal. In advanced countries like the US, the most widespread cause of death is coronary heart disease. Usage of saturated fats, bad lifestyle, and smoking, are primary causes of heightened cholesterol and its subsequent dangers.

Many drugs are now available all over the world to decrease cholesterol levels. Reductase inhibitors like HMG-CoA or better known as statins, are the most popular drugs available in the market today. This group of drugs is marketed under various brand names and helps in greatly lowering cholesterol levels in patients with high risk. They also help in increasing HDL or the 'good cholesterol'.

Even though these drugs have been proven to be effective, many people prefer not to use them and opt for alternative methods. One such method is leading an active life. Exercise and physical activity form an integral part of many therapies for low cholesterol. This results in reduction in weight, lowering of blood pressure and also greatly reduces risk of diabetes.

A proper diet with low cholesterol content can also greatly lower cholesterol levels. A good and healthy diet contains low levels of 'bad cholesterol' but sufficient quantities of 'good cholesterol'. Such a diet can lower cholesterol levels up to 29 percent in just one month's time. Therefore proper diet, just like drugs, can be effectively used for controlling cholesterol levels. Eating foods with high fibre content can reduce levels of cholesterol by almost 7 percent.

The risk of various heart diseases can be greatly reduced by using unprocessed or non-hydrogenated fats, nuts, soy proteins, barley and oats. Fish and some plant sources containing Omega-3 fats also help as do fruits and green leafy vegetables.

‍ॐ‍

CHOLESTEROL DRUGS
The Dangers

When it comes to treating high cholesterol, doctors prescribe certain drugs called statins. Formally referred to as pharmaceuticals, Statins are a specific class of drugs used to reduce cholesterol levels. There are many issues raised against the use of statin drugs and their dangers, which include: peripheral neuropathy, muscle damage, elevated liver enzyme indices, plasma fibrinogen levels and kidney damage.

You must remember however, that these are only concerns at this point in our understanding of them and not proven facts. The medical community as a whole has yet to make any definitive judgment on the allegations that are not fully corroborated studies. Some of the common side-effects which patients complain of include memory loss, personality changes, irritability and muscle pain. These do not occur in all patients but have been known to affect some.

There are seven statin drugs on the market. Those in the fermentation group are:
- lovastatin,
- pravastatin
- simvastatin

Next there are those that are in the synthetic group:
- atorvastatin
- fluvastatin
- rusovastatin
- cerivastatin

Some of the brand names of these same drugs are:

- Zocor
- Lipitor
- Pravachol

Those in the fermentation group seem to be more effective in lowering LDL levels.

Without question there have been a number of deaths that have been related to the use of statin drugs. Separating fact from speculation is however, a job for the experts. As laypeople, it is necessary to do more than simply read what the media reports on the deaths that are related to any specific medication. The media are journalists and newscasters and it is not their job to diagnose the causes of deaths. They are not medical specialists either and not equipped to do so. To better understand the real dangers of statin drug and the implications for you, consult your physician and assess the chances of major side-effects.

If you do feel that you would benefit from using any of the drugs mentioned here for controlling your cholesterol levels, your doctor is your first place to go. Follow your physician's instructions to the letter. Misusing your medication can be fatal. You should also keep following your diet and exercise plan because the drugs can only do so much to help you. In the end, you have to help yourself too.

৪৩৫৩

CHOLESTEROL REDUCING VITAMINS & DRUGS
3 Key Variations

Cholesterol is the name that scares one and all in terms of health. The key cause of heart diseases as doctors suggest, is cholesterol. High cholesterol level in the blood can not only lead to heart attacks but also cause several weight problems.

Coronary Heart Disease does not appear overnight. It gradually develops with the person's growing age and sustained high amounts of blood cholesterol. In order to live a healthy and long life it is essential to lower cholesterol levels as early as possible. Here are some specialized medications and substitutes to fight back rising cholesterol levels.

1. Statins
These are specialized medications aimed at lowering cholesterol levels. Such medications are grouped in to different classes. The most common ones available in the market are HMG-CoA Inhibitors, or statins, which reduce cholesterol by blocking the enzyme HMG-CoA. Formation of this enzyme is one of the important functions in the steps involved in the conversion of fats into cholesterol. These are to date, the most effective drugs for lowing cholesterol. They have helped many people who require urgent and drastic reduction in their cholesterol levels.

2. Bile Acid Sequestrants
The human liver produces a special bile. Cholesterol lowering drugs bind with this bile. Bile is a substance that aids the digestion system in the absorption of fats into the intestines. Bile acid sequestrant

prevents the formulation of cholesterol by preventing the bile acid from digesting the fats.

3. Vitamins

Vitamins help lower the cholesterol levels. Some of these effective vitamins are as follows:

i. Vitamin B/ Niacin

Vitamin B3 or Niacin, is the most common cholesterol lowering vitamin. It is one among the 8 water-soluble B vitamins and helps the body in the conversion of carbohydrates into glucose, which provides energy. B vitamins are also important in breaking down body fats as well as proteins and acids, which aid in making the nervous system, eyes, skin, mouth, hair and liver healthy. Niacin is also helpful in getting rid of toxic and harmful chemicals from the body.

Niacin increases the effects of other cholesterol reducing drugs as well, but only if taken in very high doses. But this is something which is not advisable, as taking large amounts of Vitamin B can lead to flushing of the skin which happens due to the dilation of blood vessels. Other side-effects of excessive intake of Vitamin B are headaches, itching, muscle cramps and nausea.

ii. Lecithin

Lecithin is among the other substances and vitamins that lower cholesterol. It allows cholesterol and fats to be eliminated from the body. It also prevents the fatty build up in the arteries.

iii. Vitamins C & E

Vitamins C & E prevent LDL cholesterol from damage, hence saving people from heart disease. While LDL cholesterol known to be the bad guy, cardiologists believe that only damaged LDL cholesterol contributes to the risk of heart diseases.

৪০৫৪

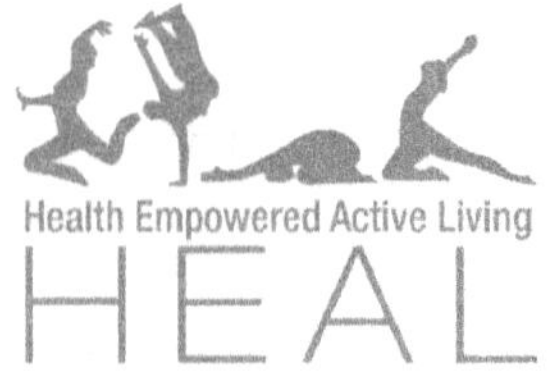
Health Empowered Active Living
HEAL

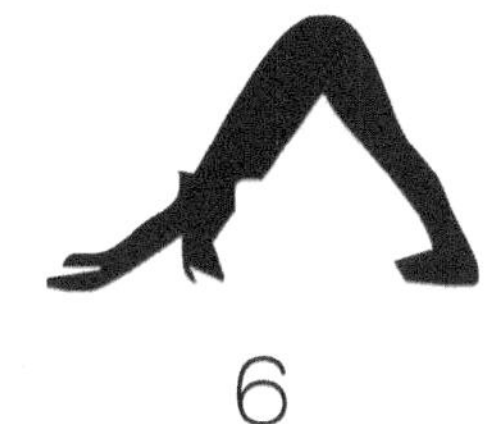

6

EXERCISE & CHOLESTEROL

LOWER CHOLESTEROL
WITH EXERCISE
14 Reasons & Tips

High cholesterol level not only leads to coronary heart disease but also several weight problems. Studies show that people with low cholesterol levels are less likely to suffer from these risks and ailments. Hence, lowering the bad cholesterol in your bloodstream is both a necessary preventive and a solution to coronary heart diseases.

Unhealthy eating and drinking habits such as extra consumption of alcohol, sugar, fats and oils can cause irreparable harm. The better way out is in that old saying, 'Prevention is better that cure'. The need is to change our lifestyle and add the little habits that help us live longer, healthier and happier. These changes are often hard to make and even harder to sustain, calling for both sacrifices and adjustments, but ultimately they pay off in terms of good health. It is important to act early and quickly as ageing is another factor that adds to cholesterol related problems. The younger one is, the easier it is to sustain the changes and avoid the ill effects.

Here are some easy tips to use in your daily life.

1.   Eat a controlled diet, preferably prescribed by a professional dietician.

2.   Exercising is the healthiest of all resorts against cholesterol and the most effective as well in the long run.

3. Exercising increases the heart rate and improves the metabolism of the body, allowing improved expulsion of harmful oils which are detrimental to health.

4. What exercise or what type of exercises to do depends on various factors, along with one's medical history. The deciding factors also include age, gender and weight.

5. For those who are new to an exercise regimen, it is advisable to first consult a physician and check out what is safe and what is not in their particular case.

6. Those already suffering with heart trouble may be advised against particular rigorous exercises. In such cases simpler alternates are often advised, such as stretching, weight lifting, walking, etc.

7. In case your physician allows you to participate in high impact exercises, try swimming, running, bicycling, aerobics, etc.

8. Ask your doctor to sketch your fitness plan in detail and stick to it with the guidance of a professional fitness trainer. As a good patient and a responsible individual, following the plan is in your hands.

9. Usually the results of such plans become evident within a week or two. Soon the bad cholesterol starts reducing and being replaced with good cholesterol, leading to a considerable reduction in body weight as well.

10. Exercising is considered the best resort as it has few or no side-effects.

11. In case you do not have time in your daily schedule to go to a gym, try a simple, brisk walk in the early morning or before going to your workplace.

12. Some organizations encourage their people to walk up 1 or 2 flights of stairs, instead of using the elevator. Try it. It is a good habit.

13. Where companies have large parking lots, a walking track around the area would be of great benefit. Walking a few yards will make a lot of difference.

14. Whenever taking up any exercise, consuming plenty of water will helps a great deal. This prevents the body from becoming dehydrated and repercussions like exhaustion. To keep hydrated, you do not have to keep running to the water fountain, just carry a water bottle with you. While working also, especially in a group activity, this simple thing really helps when moving from your place repeatedly would not be considered professional.

ಶುಭ